Lose Weight This Way

Not That Way

Lose weight without dieting, even while you sleep and keep it off forever

Kristine Knutson M.D

INTRODUCTION

CHAPTER ONE

THE WRONG WEIGHTLOSS APPROACH

CHAPTER TWO

WEIGHTLOSS AND YOUR BODY TYPE
Hire a detective

CHAPTER THREE

WEIGHT LOSS AND DIET
Emotional Eating

CHAPTER FOUR

WEIGHT LOSS AND DEPRESSION

CHAPTER FIVE

WEIGHT LOSS AND ANXIETY

CHAPTER SIX

WEIGHT LOSS & STRESS

CHAPTER SEVEN

CHOCOLATE AND YOUR MOOD
Do you love chocolate and sweets?
Low serotonin levels

CHAPTER EIGHT

WEIGHT LOSS AND WILL POWER

CHAPTER NINE

WEIGHT LOSS AND THE DRIVE
Know your motivation keys

CHAPTER TEN

Lose Weight This Way Not That Way

INTRODUCTION

Have you tried to lose weight but failed time and time again?

One key reason weight loss effort fails is because people think of it at a superficial level.

This book will help you look at the complete picture instead of focusing on just a part.

You will get to the root of the challenge, so you have complete information on how to solve it.

That way, you will see how to approach food from a nutrition/health perspective and not just from a weight gain/ weight loss perspective.

You will learn about your body, its makeup, and how best to work with it.

There are three body types; you will know your type, and what is appropriate for it so you can lose the extra pounds and look and feel your best.

This way, you will know it is futile to do what other people are doing because your body type and theirs are not the same.

This book will show you methods that work well and fast for whatever body type you have.

You will learn all you need to know, so you lose weight and don't gain it back.

CHAPTER ONE

THE WRONG WEIGHTLOSS APPROACH

There was a scenario that happened one day; Alexa left home without knowing that she didn't turn off one of the taps before leaving the house.

When she came back from work, she discovered there was water everywhere. Water had soaked the furniture and other things.

Shocked at the sight, she hurriedly got a small bucket and a mug and then started fetching water from the floor into the bucket.

Now pause!

Is Alexa missing something here?

Yes.

She is busy – yea!

She is taking water from the room to outside the house – yea!

But she is yet to solve the problem at the root; unless she turns off that running tap, she would mop water for a long time.

As long as she is working the mug and bucket, the problem will persist?

Many people are like Alexa; they run to the latest fad that promises them weight loss without first turning off the tap.

CHAPTER TWO

WEIGHTLOSS AND YOUR BODY TYPE

When it comes to our bodies, it's not the same, we have different body types, and this difference matters when it comes to nutrition, exercise, and weight loss.

Being armed with this information will help you know how to treat your body the way that fits.

The three different body types are the ectomorph, mesomorph, and endomorph.

The metabolic rate of an ectomorph is very fast, and that's why they are lean.

Even if an ectomorph gained some weight because of any other reason, they find it easy to lose this weight without making the extra effort other body types will make.

Mesomorphs have a naturally fit body even if they don't exercise. In addition, mesomorphs are less vulnerable to weight gain than endomorphs because of their high metabolism level.

Their lifestyle is usually full of action and vigorous exercises, which helps them stay in form even if they eat much.

You might have already guessed that endomorphs are the most vulnerable people to gain weight.

Their bodies are usually soft and round, and the rate at which they can lose weight is much less than that of other body types.

If you are an endomorph, then the most important advice you must remember at all times is for you not to compare yourself to others.

Going to the gym with a mesomorph friend may cause you disappointment when they start getting in shape faster than you.

On the other hand, comparing yourself to an ectomorph will surely disappoint you because weight loss is pretty easy for them.

As an endomorph, you can gain muscles that replace fat easier than the ectomorph, ensure your diet is more of proteins than carbohydrates, and you need regular exercise.

So endomorph also has something others don't have. I think that's great.

Being an endomorph means that your metabolic rate is a bit slow. Therefore, you can't depend on diet alone for weight loss.

Ensure you adopt the eating habits prescribed in this book and follow the other instructions mentioned in this book.

The important thing you must note that people can fit somewhere between two body types; for example, if you are in between the endomorph and the mesomorph, then gaining some muscles while losing fat will give you the perfect body.

Hire a detective

What will happen if someone you don't know hires the best spy CIA or Mossad agent to gather information on you?

That spy would track when you wake and go to sleep, how much time you sit per day, your usual route to anywhere and back home, your activity level, the time you spent online, etc.

The agent will follow you around for, say, 30 – 60 days, and guess what happens.

They will collate this information and then predict your future behavior.

And they will be mostly right because they see the pattern of your habits and habits are quite reliable in predicting people, whether these habits are soft or hard.

What if this agent was you?

Would that make any difference?

It would make a world of difference.

There are recurring commands you follow that you have not taken time to pause and examine for once.

There are beliefs you have rehearsed, live, and acted that you have not questioned for once.

Two things I want to recommend as you take this weight loss journey.

Get a journal and a scale.

With the journal, you will write down the food you consume and you will use the scale to know your weight.

Fill in the foods you consume for breakfast, lunch, and dinner. Don't judge yourself as you do this exercise. Just live your life but record this aspect of your life for four weeks.

Every morning get on a scale and record your weight.

Write down the number, again calmly speak to yourself not to throw judgment but to show self-compassion.

Talk to yourself comas if there is another self that can hear you.

Research shows that one of the under-reported secrets to weight loss is journaling.

When you can keep record of your food and weight consistently every day for the next four weeks, you will be able to change your life.

Whatever you do, complete the four weeks of recording your food and weight every single day.

Can you do that?

Just that.

No exercise.

No diet pills.

No nothing.

Just record. Period!

We have established a background for what will help you overcome the challenge of extra weight.

Let's take a look at your motivations or drive as to why you want to lose weight.

Your motivation will determine if you will succeed or fail, but I am here to ensure you don't fail.

Kristine Knutson

CHAPTER THREE

WEIGHT LOSS AND DIET

How many times have you attempted to diet and failed?

How many times have you suffered the pain of not eating what you want and then ended up with no result?

Like the story of Alexa, where she was busy mopping water instead of first turning off the tap, in the same way, many people approach their weight loss issue.

If you are serious about losing weight, you should detect the root cause of your eating habits and other factors that may contribute.

Most times, diet doesn't work because it does not address the root problem.

You can use diet alongside other techniques to remove the main culprit that leads to emotional eating.

Or would you be ready to stick to the painful alternative of dieting for the rest of your life?

Emotional Eating

Whenever we face problems in life and whenever circumstances become intolerable, we try to find a way to escape from the pain.

The problem is that you are escaping to feel better by indulging habits that may not be good for your health.

For example, if you observe the people who smoke, they smoke when certain conditions are right. Like, when they are:

- stressed
- anxious
- frustrated

- unsatisfied
- uncomfortable

As you can see, I have listed many reasons that are not related to the cigarette itself or nicotine addiction but have everything to do with one's mood.

These people usually use their cigarettes to escape unwanted emotions, and they may not even be aware of that.

They may be thinking that they can't stop smoking because of nicotine addiction or lack of willpower, but the truth is people smoke because they seek to escape.

Everyone has his way of escaping. Some smoke, some others eat food for comfort, others go back to their ex or seek a new relationship, some escape to drugs.

Unfortunately, many people are obese not because of their genes or body type but because they escape to food whenever they have bad moods.

Two problems arise from this escaping unwanted emotions.

The first is that your real problems are never solved, and the second is that you gain weight and become obese.

What makes emotional eating much more dangerous is that most people are unaware they are eating to escape, but they tell themselves they eat because it tastes delicious.

The other thing is, life is full of problems and ups and downs, and if you built the habit of eating whenever you felt like escaping distressing emotions, you would find yourself eating here and there with no self-control.

Our emotions may change many times throughout the day, and mood swings come unannounced.

Imagine yourself having a meal whenever your moods are low? How can a diet ever help such a person?

It will never help because it does not address the real problem, and it interferes with your escape method.

How can you get over your emotional eating?

As you may have already guessed, cutting the root is the solution to solving real problems.

I know what you might be thinking right now; you're probably asking yourself if it was possible to solve all your problems or even prevent yourself from feeling bad.

If you could do this, you would have done it earlier for the sake of being happy.

I am not asking you to solve these problems today, but I am just asking you to learn how to cope with those problems that can't be solved and solve the ones that you can solve.

For example, prolonged stress can lead to depression. I know that sometimes life can be stressful, and you may not be able to change the source(s) of stress, but you can learn how to change your response to the stimulus instead of changing the stimulus itself?

Stress management, anger management, and coping techniques are all methods that can help you in changing your response to an event.

Imagine if you learned how to cope with stress more effectively. Do you know how different your life would be?

Surely stressful events will still be there, but your response to them will differ, and you would feel less stressed.

It will, in turn, result in less emotional eating and will be reflected in your body shape.

Please write down the unwanted emotions you want to deal with and learn how to deal with them; only then can your emotional eating habit change.

The other thing is, your subconscious mind doesn't know of a better way to communicate with you other than sending you some emotions.

Your subconscious mind doesn't send you stress, anger, sadness, or even depression for no reason, but it's just its way of informing you that something is wrong.

Sending you emotions is its way of getting your attention and spurring you to take action.

Now suppose that you went to eat whenever you got one of these messages; what do you think your subconscious mind will do?

It will resend the signal, but this time with a stronger intensity since you didn't respond to the first signal correctly.

You would feel twice as bad or twice as stressed because you didn't respond correctly to the previous signal.

A reinforcing cycle is created because the subconscious mind perceives that you didn't respond to its messages, and the result is some extra pounds.

The great thing about these signals is that they are withdrawn as soon as you start taking action and not when you solve the problem.

I'm sure overeating had caused you to feel guilty before and realized that you felt far better as soon as you started a diet program.

In this case, the guilt was nothing but a signal from your subconscious mind asking you to change your eating habits.

When you responded to its signal, your subconscious mind decided that there was no use of the signal and finally stopped sending it.

If you take action and the signal is still there, be aware that your subconscious mind does not trust your action.

In the diet example, if this was your 12th diet program, then the signal may not be removed because the subconscious mind, in this case, doesn't think that starting a diet again would be something effective.

To summarize this part in a few words, the only way to deal with emotional eating is to solve problems that can be solved and cope with the ones you can't solve.

CHAPTER FOUR

WEIGHT LOSS AND DEPRESSION

I am quite certain you must have noticed how many depressed people either loss or gain weight in a significant manner.

Depression can influence a person's appetite and eating behavior, and that's why you can observe remarkable changes in someone's physical appearance after experiencing depression for some time.

It turns out bad when obese people face depression and experience a sudden change in their eating habits, letting them eat more.

Research has shown that weight problems can lead to depression; in this case, the person's concern about his self-image and physical looks leads to becoming depressed.

You may have already concluded how troubling that is if obesity can lead to depression.

And depression, in turn, can result in gaining additional weight, then this could result in the creation of a self-reinforcing cycle of depression and overeating.

The question you should be asking yourself is, am I depressed? And if your answer was yes, then you should ask yourself another question, is my depression responsible for my eating habits?

Even if you were not so sure, you have to know that depression can be one of the root causes for your extra weight.

Again, don't escape from depression by eating but instead try to seek help to prevent this infinite loop of eating and depression that eventually leads to changing your physical look.

CHAPTER FIVE

WEIGHT LOSS AND ANXIETY

One other emotion that can give a boost to your appetite is anxiety. Anxiety can overstimulate the systems in your body and thus increase your hunger without a real need for food.

Life is full of uncertainties, and facing situations that make us anxious is very likely to happen many times throughout the day.

What do you think will happen if every time you felt anxious, you ate more than your body needs? And what if eating became your preferred escape method whenever you felt anxious?

After all, you may be gaining weight because of your poor anxiety handling skills and not because of your love for food.

I know that you like to eat and that food tastes good, but how many times do you eat to escape from a certain unwanted emotion and not because you were really in need of food?

Some people gain extra weight during exams, not only because they spend lots of time sitting but also because of the bad mood they experience that makes them eat even if they were not feeling hungry.

Learning how to deal with anxiety and life uncertainties will remove one other item from your list of things that trigger emotional eating.

Kristine Knutson

CHAPTER SIX

WEIGHT LOSS & STRESS

Life in the twenty-first century can be very stressful; people keep going round in circles when they wake up until they go to sleep.

Some people even carry their stress into their beds, thinking about their jobs and other problems before they sleep.

Continuous stress results in sustaining high cortisol levels (otherwise known as the stress hormone), leading to adrenal fatigue.

The adrenal glands become exhausted and unable to produce adequate hormones. Adrenal fatigue results in food cravings and thus leads to overeating.

In addition to this, the high levels of cortisol that result from chronic stress were found to decrease muscle tissues. Since muscle tissues burn more calories at rest than other tissues, the decrease of muscle tissues results in weight gain.

Stress is also one factor that depletes the hormone serotonin, a hormone responsible for making you feel good. When the serotonin level depletes, you start craving carbohydrates and sugars to restore those serotonin levels to their original level.

That's why many people working under stressful conditions for a long time have fat accumulations in their bodies.

There are lots of natural ways that can help increase serotonin production and thus hinder unhelpful eating habits. On the next page, you will find more information on serotonin and the factors that affect its production.

You could be doing everything by the book but still are gaining weight because of your high-stress level. Combating stress should be one of your priorities because stress can increase your weight and cause other serious health issues.

CHAPTER SEVEN

CHOCOLATE AND YOUR MOOD

Do you love chocolate and sweets?

Chocolate and sweets contain sugar that raises the level of the hormone serotonin in your blood.

Serotonin is sometimes called the happiness hormone because it's the hormone that helps in combating depression, lifting your mood, and making you feel happy.

Some people eat chocolate to balance their serotonin levels. Unfortunately, these people are usually unaware that they are eating chocolate to balance their hormones and not because they want it.

These people don't just love chocolate, but they need it. How many times have you eaten chocolate because you were feeling bad? And how many times have you used chocolate to regulate your mood or to feel better?

Becoming aware of your eating habits' real reasons will help you lose weight and understand yourself more.

Next time you decided to bite out of this delicious dessert, ask yourself one question, do I love it, or do I need it to appease my mood?

Low serotonin levels

Carbohydrates increase the serotonin level in your blood, thus changing your mood for the better. That's why some people start eating when they feel bad.

It's crucial to realize whether you are eating to raise your serotonin level or because you are hungry.

Once you feel that you are eating to feel better, you probably should understand that the problem is with your body's hormones and not your need for food.

Don't worry; there are lots of natural ways that increase your serotonin level other than eating, such as:

Exposure to direct sunlight increases serotonin levels. That's why few minutes of being in the sun perceptibly improve your mood; this happens because serotonin is produced in the presence of sunlight?

Vitamins like B and C play a role in serotonin production.

Ensure your diet includes those vitamins. You don't have to eat an apple pie to feel good; some fruits will be a better replacement.

Exercising increases serotonin's natural levels. If you don't play any sports consider running at the very least.

As you can see, your lifestyle can affect your serotonin levels. For example, if you wake up late, miss the sunlight and never exercise, then no wonder you will find yourself feeling bad most of the time.

Slight changes to your daily activities can affect your serotonin production and so affect your mood. So waking up a bit earlier, catching the sunlight, and exercising will surely help you feel better. So you won't be dependent on food to change your mood.

Lose Weight This Way Not That Way

CHAPTER EIGHT

WEIGHT LOSS AND WILL POWER

Like most people, you have tried to use willpower to stop binge eating, but it never works regardless of your best intentions.

The problem is that willpower is not a reliable source of motivation unless you tweak something.

Here is why willpower does not work naturally.

Let's imagine that you had a good day and were happy; you are very likely to resist the urge to eat your favorite food in such an emotional state.

Still, if something upsets your mood, you'll most likely discover that you will struggle to resist.

Will power changes along with your mood, and that's why depending on willpower alone to stop bad habits will never work.

Will power will only help you as long as you feel good, but it may fail to help you when your mood swings.

So the question is, how do I break the habit of overeating? There are two types of motivation styles that people respond to, which are positive and negative.

Some people are mostly motivated by rewards, they respond to positive motivation, while those motivated by the desire to avoid punishment respond to negative motivation.

So how can you make use of these motivation styles to motivate yourself to stop eating?

First of all, you must understand the effect of visualization on your motivation levels. Visualization is what you see with your eyes or with your mind's eyes.

Your subconscious mind responds to the images and things you see, which flows into mental impressions, mood fluctuation, and how you act without thinking about it.

Just observe how you act when seeing a horror movie. You will find that your body is triggering the fight and flight response.

It is preparing itself from running from some perceived danger even when you are in a familiar environment like your home.

If you tried to monitor your thoughts, you would find that you visualize the food in your mind before going to the refrigerator or the kitchen.

Visualisation of the food leads to a craving to eat.

Some people even become hungry due to visualizing a specific food or treat and not because their bodies need any food.

Visualization motivates the subconscious mind to trigger hunger to respond to its cue via the images seen.

The long and short story is that images or videos can program your subconscious mind. Visualization could help you take action or break a habit.

Now let's combine both forms of motivation.

Search the web and find an image of someone having the perfect body, searching for another image of a very obese person you never want to be.

Now use any image editor to put those two pictures together as one image (the picture of the obese person should be next to the picture of your dream body).

Next, remove the faces with an image editor and put your face instead, as this would bring the point home.

Now you have an image that provides you with both positive and negative motivation. All you have to do is make copies and place them everywhere in your space and let your subconscious mind do the rest.

Here are the places you should put that image:

- make it your desktop wallpaper
- make it your mobile phone background image
- place it on the walls in your house
- hang it in on the door of your room
- set it above your bed
- place it on your desk
- put it in front of you while eating (if you still catch yourself binge eating)
- finally, above your television

Every time you see this picture, your subconscious mind will become more motivated to be like the preferable body.

It will become more motivated to stay away from the habits that could lead to being similar to the other image.

You have just combined motivation and visualization concepts in one step by just investing one hour of your time preparing these pictures.

CHAPTER NINE

WEIGHT LOSS AND THE DRIVE

People often fail to break bad habits because they lack a strong drive.

It means that if you had a powerful drive not to binge eat, you would never do it.

Suppose you were trapped in a room full of your favorite food and that you were starving. You saw something disgusting in the food, maybe some dead rat, or you learn that the food had been poisoned right after taking the first bite of the food.

Would you continue to eat this food even if you were starving?

The chances are high that you would stop eating because the drive motivating you to stop is very strong, your desire to live or your disgust.

On the other hand, if you were at home and could smell your favorite food, you are more likely to eat it than in the previous case.

The conclusion is if you can find a strong drive that can prevent you from eating, then use it.

The pictures you got from the internet in the previous section can help you increase such a drive.

You can also use obesity health risk conditions to increase your drive if you care about your health.

Here are some obesity health risks conditions:

Physical health risks

- increases the risk of a heart disease

- increases risk of strokes
- hypertension is more common among obese people
- aches and pain that result from the stress on muscles and joints
- increases risk of type 2 diabetes
- increases risk of colon and gall balder cancer
- infertility

Psychological health risks

- poor self-image
- low self-esteem
- depression
- again putting such a list everywhere in your home can dramatically increase your motivation to lose weight.

Know your motivation keys

One essential thing you should notice is that not everyone will be motivated by seeing the same things.

Every person has got his/her motivation keys.

Understanding your keys won't be a challenging task. But, first, try to identify the things that you value most or the things you want most.

Do you want to have more self-confidence?

Are you obsessed with your body image?

Do you want to live a healthy life while avoiding diseases?

Do you have an identity you cherish so much?

Understanding your needs will guide you to the things you need to do to motivate yourself.

For example, suppose you are very concerned about your physical appearance more than anything else.

In that case, the picture of the obese and slim guy we talked about earlier will be your best method.

Find that thing that motivates you the most, then put a picture of this motive everywhere.

When criticism becomes the drive

Some people only start to think about losing weight when they get criticized for their looks by others.

Had they not received such comments, they would have left themselves without taking any action.

If this is the case, I suggest using the drive concept we talked about earlier to motivate yourself other than people's criticism.

Why wait until someone hurts you?

And why be a reactive person who only acts when it's too late?

Why not be a proactive person who takes action just before the problem happens?

Finding a new drive or identity that can motivate you won't be challenging, but leaving yourself to the mercy of these comments will only make your life miserable.

You will only be alerted when it's too late.

Other people only start a diet because they are concerned about their looks in the swimming suit. Those people usually stop the diet as soon as the summer is over.

If you think like that, then you don't value yourself as you might like to think.

If you don't act in ways that show that you value yourself and make every effort to be healthy, you will lack self-confidence.

You will only become confident when you treat yourself well and prove to your subconscious mind that you are worthy.

By taking care of your looks for the sole reason of getting other people's approval, you tell your subconscious mind that you are worthless and that what matters is other people's opinions.

You're also telling your subconscious mind that making others happy by providing them with what they want (seeing you take a particular shape) is more important than your wants or needs.

In this case, the price you are paying to get their approval is at the expense of your self-confidence.

Taking care of yourself and your looks should be part of your lifestyle (your identity, not just a goal) and not just something you do whenever the summer approaches.

Suppose its criticism that motivates you to stop eating or to exercise.

In that case, we can use that drive differently, get a journal, and record the worst comments and criticism that have been directed at you about your weight.

You should use this journal the same way I explained you use that picture mentioned in an earlier section; all you have to do is make copies and put this journal within your line of vision to see it now and then at different places.

In this case, you are using a negative motivation to motivate yourself; negative motivation can be compelling but at a price.

It continually reminds you of the things you hate, which could make you feel bad.

Just ask yourself one question, why do I feel bad when I read these remarks? Is it because the people who gave these remarks were rude, or is it because they are a constant reminder of my lack of responsibility?

People usually feel bad upon being reminded of their obesity when they're not doing anything about it, when they're not giving their all to lose the extra weight. If you're doing your best, then there's no way the criticism will be that painful.

The comments only get to you because they remind you of what you're trying to escape; you don't feel bad because of their remarks, but because of the guilt you feel when you realize how badly you are treating your body.

You feel bad because you are forced to face the truth that you still have to make more effort to achieve the right image.

These critics are not to be blamed because it's your escaping the problem that got you to feel bad; all they did was remind you.

Make sure you keep recording whatever you consume and your weight every day.

Don't stop that activity for anything. The other exercises mentioned in this book are not to replace them but to complement them.

CHAPTER TEN

WEIGHT LOSS AND YOUR METABOLISM

Your body was designed for survival and not for modeling.

All the vital functions inside your body serve one purpose, which is preventing you from dying.

What do you think will happen if you didn't eat for 10 hours intentionally?

What will happen is that your body will reduce the consumption of the food it takes by slowing down your metabolic rate.

Unfortunately, it means that preventing yourself from eating can result in weight gain and not weight loss in the long term.

After all, the faster your metabolic rate, the faster the rate of burning fats.

People who undergo strict diets could gain weight if they did it the incorrect way. Contrary to common beliefs, the more meals you eat (without eating in-between), the faster your metabolic rate.

For example, eating five small meals a day will prevent you from feeling hungry and, at the same will increase your metabolic rate as opposed to eating three big meals where you are more likely to gain weight.

Research shows that people who ate breakfast regularly weighed less than those who didn't.

It happens because of the same survival concept, and your body wakes up in need of energy. Still, when it doesn't find any, it slows down its metabolic rate to preserve some of the existing energy, resulting in weight gain.

Metabolic rate and muscles

Studies report that lean muscle tissues require more calories to sustain themselves even if you aren't making any effort.

It means that people who have more lean muscle tissue lose more calories than others even if they are at rest.

What's excellent about lean muscle tissues is that they can be developed. Strength training can help you develop more lean muscle tissues and, in turn, speed up your metabolism, leading you to lose more weight.

One other thing that can boost your metabolic rate is exercising regularly. Unfortunately, people think of exercising as a fast method to change their body shape, and as soon as they lose some pounds, they stop training.

You don't need to guess what will happen to them; they will regain the lost weight.

That's why I mentioned at the beginning of the book that maintaining a healthy weight is more dependent on your lifestyle and not on the short-term diet programs that you follow.

A diet program can make you lose weight, but your lifestyle will bring back the lost pounds. This point should let you look at exercising from another perspective.

Exercising should be viewed to increase your metabolic rate so long as you are doing it. So exercising is a habit that you should develop and make a permanent part of your lifestyle.

You don't have to lift weights or do vigorous exercise. Just commit to walking or running for 15 hours a day. The reason exercising doesn't work for most people is that:

- They usually do it for a short period then stop
- They only start exercising when they find that they need to lose weight.

Some start exercising at the end of April (because the summer is approaching) then quit a few months later

Exercising should become a habit and not just a fast method of removing some extra pounds.

Women tend to ignore strength training, thinking that it's guys' stuff, which is not correct.

No one said that you should lift as heavyweights as men do; a few minutes of strength training every week will surely help you burn fats much faster.

In addition, men tend to lose weight faster than women because of their additional muscle tissues, which require more calories to sustain.

So, as a woman, you should consider building some muscle tissues to increase your metabolic rate (calorie-burning speed), which will, in turn, help you lose weight faster.

Tea & your metabolic rate

Drinking tea is another natural way to increase your metabolic rate. The caffeine found in tea helps the body to burn more calories and to increase its metabolic rate.

For example, suppose you can drink tea after each meal (but give yourself one hour first to digest food because tea can prevent iron absorption). In that case, you will find that food intake is not affecting you as it always used to do.

Green tea is even better because it has the same benefits, only healthier. Green tea is a natural, safe way of burning fats and increasing the metabolic rate. In addition to that, it prevents your blood sugar levels from rising that much after a meal.

You can send me a mail to recommend a green tea brand for best result drkristineknuston@gmail.com

Again, you should not drink green tea for few days then quit when you feel like wanting to quit, but it should be a part of your new lifestyle.

Alcohol and your metabolic rate

Up till now, I haven't found a health problem that hasn't got alcohol consumption related to its development.

The same goes for overeating; alcohol consumption alone can't increase your weight, but it does stimulate your appetite to eat more.

I know there are times when drinking alcohol is unavoidable but consider it as a challenge to how much you want to lose weight.

So, again, I'll ask the very same question: do you want to lose weight?

If you do, why do you keep stuff that hinders your ability to control your eating habits?

Our society may have led us to believe that losing weight is a complicated process, but it's only those who want to lose it who do.

What I meant by the word "want" is the powerful desire of really wanting to do something; it's that power that stops you from any act that might stand in the way of achieving your goals.

Some people want to lose weight, while others dream of losing weight. Those who want to lose weight are the ones who keep applying whatever they learn until something works. In contrast, the others keep blaming the whole world for their problem without taking a single step towards solving it.

Vitamins and your metabolic rate

Vitamins can help you feel more energetic, leading you to do more work and lose more calories. Vitamins also play a role in speeding up your metabolism, which results in burning more fats.

Vitamin B -12 can give you an energy boost, and thus it's helpful in weight loss. Vitamin b -12 can be found in eggs, fish, and beef.

In addition, vegetables and fruits are good sources of vitamins, and that's why it's always a good idea to replace desserts with fruits. A balanced diet is a substantial factor that can result in weight loss and a healthy body.

Ensure that your diet includes vitamins, carbohydrates, and proteins instead of just focusing on one of them.

Weight loss and eating slowly

When your body needs food, your brain starts to send you the signal of hunger so that you supply it with the nourishment it needs.

When you eat sufficient food that satisfied your body's needs, your brain withdraws this signal and sends you the sign of fullness. However, even if you ate a lot, the fullness signal won't be sent before 15 to 20 minutes after eating.

It means that if you eat very fast, you will more likely eat more food before feeling full.

In this case, your body may have already had its needed supplies, but the signal still can't be sent before the 20 minutes pass.

You can make use of this concept by eating as slow as you can. Chew food well and slow down a bit while eating, and this will result in receiving the fullness signal before you eat lots of food that your body doesn't need.

Weight loss and fibers

Fibers don't only facilitate digestion; besides, it helps you reduce the fats in your body and lose weight. Fibers are found in fruits, vegetables, and whole grains.

Fibers can make you feel full sooner than other types of food. They also stay longer in your stomach and so you feel full for a more extended time.

Ensuring that your meal has the right amount of fiber will make you full without consuming the same calories as before.

Fibers don't contain any calories or fat, and that's why eating large amounts of fiber can never increase your weight.

Fibers also help in moving fats faster through the digestive system and thus resulting in making you slimmer.

A good trick is to start your meal with a green salad.

After you finish it, you can then move on to the rest of the food.

By doing so, you are making yourself feel full before you even start eating calorie-rich food.

Another good thing you can do is replacing desserts with fruits. And if you were dying for a dessert, you can first eat some fruits then go for the desert; this may result in finding yourself full and thus ignoring the desert. Even if you eat a small portion, the fruits will prevent you from eating a larger amount by filling a part of your stomach.

Weight loss and protein intake

Research has found that eating protein could dampen your hunger to a certain extent. When you start eating, try to begin by eating proteins first to feel a bit full before eating other food types to increase your weight.

Protein is also harder to digest than carbohydrates, resulting in feeling full for a more extended time and eating less.

I have previously mentioned that lean muscles consume more energy than other cells. So it is another reason why protein can help in weight loss because it helps develop muscles (if accompanied by regular exercising).

Protein helps produce glucagon, a hormone that can help the body get rid of fats. So contrary to eating carbohydrates which may result in insulin resistance (where your body ignores the effect of insulin and stores fats instead of getting rid of them), protein helps produce insulin that further supports weight loss.

Beware that too much protein can be dangerous to your kidneys and internal organs. The key is to use protein as a method of feeling full rather than increasing its intake.

High-calorie intake leads to more weight

The more calories you eat, the more likely you will want to eat again.

Research has found that eating a meal that contains high calories may trigger your hunger again faster than what would have happened if your dinner included fewer calories.

In an experiment lab, rats were divided into two groups, the first group was fed a high-fat diet, and the second group was fed a low-fat diet.

After that, the researcher introduced a fatty meal to both groups, and the first group ate more than the second group.

The same could happen to you, just as with the rats. Studies find that obese people always report that they are not satisfied with their meals and demand larger food amounts.

The hormone leptin increases in your blood whenever it finds that fat is accumulating. Leptin is the hormone responsible for reducing your body fats, and it's sometimes called the slimming hormone.

So the more fat you have, the higher the leptin level in your blood and the faster you will lose weight, right?

That's not right because leptin levels bypass a specific limit; the brain tends to ignore leptin resistance. But, again, this does mean that the more fats you accumulate by eating foods with a high level of fats, the more you will gain weight because of leptin resistance.

Again I am not asking you to stop eating your favorite food but you should consider eating less of the foods that contain high fats and eating more of the foods that contain low fats. The following is an example of types of food that have high fat levels:

- French fries
- Milk shakes
- Beef & pork
- Turkey
- Chicken
- Chocolate
- Chicken pot pie
- Pie
- Condensed milk
- Cheesecake
- Meat hamburgers and cheeseburgers
- Tacos & nachos
- Chicken fillet sandwiches
- Eggs
- Bacon
- Onion rings

In addition to this, your body needs more energy to convert carbohydrates into fats than that it needs to convert high-fat food into fats.

The preceding sentence means that out of each 1000 calories of carbohydrates you consume, more calories are required to convert these 1000 calories into fats than the calories needed to convert high-fat food into fats.

Suppose we assumed that your body needs around 100 calories to store those 1000. In that case, you are bringing in 900 calories to your body (1000-100). In high-fat foods, the energy needed will be much less than these 100 calories to be more weight.

High carbohydrates lead to more eating.

When you eat high carbohydrates, insulin is released to relocate the sugar in the blood and take it to the cells that need it.

It is a healthy system, but if the insulin level keeps surging now and then due to a high-carb diet, the cells' response will be less sensitive to insulin. That results in preventing the adequate amount of glucose from reaching the cells, leading to cravings of carbohydrates, leading to overeating and weight gain.

The overconsumption of simple carbohydrates can give you a burst of energy for a few hours. However, the downside is that as your insulin level increases and the effect of these simple sugars goes away, your blood sugar level will suddenly drop and trigger the brain to send hunger signals again.

Thus, it results in a self-reinforcing cycle of simple craving carbohydrates and eating while ultimately leads to weight gain.

It should be clear now that it's only us fooling ourselves when we say something like: "I will only eat that piece and nothing more" or when we say something like: "I will only take a small bite of that cake then I won't get near it again.

As you can see, the more carbohydrates you eat, the more you will crave additional portions and the more weight you will gain; high food intake leads to other cravings, which leads to increased food intake.

To overcome this problem and break this cycle, you must shift from high-carb diets to balanced diets that contain equal portions of all types of food.

Water and weight loss

Water can help you in burning your calories and in fuelling your metabolism. What's good about water is that it can make you feel full, and there are no health risks associated with drinking lots of it.

Studies have shown that staying dehydrated could result in fat accumulation. On the other hand, giving your body an adequate water supply can help reduce those fats. Water helps supply your body with oxygen, which is essential in the fat-burning process; if you kept your body dehydrated, more fats would accumulate due to the burning process's slowdown.

A research proved that drinking from long thin glasses results in drinking less than in short wide glasses. It is because people tend to notice height more than width, and that's why replacing your short glasses with tall ones will make you drink less juice or fizzy drinks.

When the body is adequately hydrated, the kidneys function properly; thus, the kidneys do not function correctly without water.

The body delegates some of the kidneys' tasks to the liver. The liver itself helps in weight loss through the role it plays in fat burning.

Now, what if the liver was busy doing the extra tasks assigned to it because of the water shortage? The result will be more fat accumulation and more reason to drink as much water as you can.

There is a perfect trick that you can do to prevent yourself from drinking juices full of sugar. As soon as you feel thirsty, go to the kitchen and drink water first before taking a sip of the juice you intend to consume.

Drinking one glass of water will make you feel full, and you won't find more space for the juice except for a small amount.

By doing this, you are not preventing yourself from drinking your favorite drink, and at the same time, you are making sure that you are only getting a small amount.

CHAPTER ELEVEN
WRONG SIGNAL

Some people confuse feelings of thirst with feelings of hunger!! When your body becomes dehydrated, its signals may sometimes be perceived as hunger instead of thirst.

So people go ahead and eat when it's water that their bodies want. Of course, there isn't a clue in such a situation that can help you figure out whether you're starving or not; what you can do is a small trick through which you can overcome this problem.

Whenever you feel like eating, try drinking first; if, after a few minutes, you still feel hungry, then you probably need food. You should do that even if you feel hungry, as drinking will dampen your appetite and eat less.

Some people fool themselves by drinking soda and soft drinks instead of water. But, first, you have to know that your drinking habits may be mainly contributing to your weight gain; with each glass of juice you drink, you're giving more sugars to your body and thus further triggering the cycle of additional eating and weight gain.

Controlling your drinking habits is s important as maintaining your eating habits in the process of weight loss.

Unfortunately, drinking habits could be even more dangerous because people don't feel the same amount of guilt upon drinking a glass of juice accompanied by eating a piece of cake.

However, suppose you calculate the number of calories in each cup of juice and each can of soda you drink. In that case, you'll find that you are gaining weight mostly because of the number of drinks you consume.

You might underestimate the number of calories found in a soda or some other juice; if each bottle contains something like 300 calories, then drinking three sodas a day can add around 1000 calories to your diet; consider that you haven't eaten anything yet

What if you drink five bottles a day? What if you drink more?

Again the solution for this problem is drinking water. Let drinking water be a rule that you follow whenever you want to eat or drink; as soon as you wake up, drink a glass of water and drink another as soon as you get home.

By doing so, you won't be feeling like you're depriving yourself of eating anything. At the same time, you'll be damping your appetite in a way that will help you lose weight much faster.

Weight loss and the shape of your plate

Since many psychological factors affect your appetite, you can do simple tricks to fool your body by making it think it's already full. The choice of your plate is one of the factors that can affect your feeling of fullness.

A small plate full of food will make you feel full more than a big plate that is half full. Change your plate size, and you will find that you feel full much faster than before.

In addition to the plate size, the number of plates containing food on the table can stimulate your appetite. For example, suppose your table was stuffed with different plates containing different food types.

In that case, you are more likely to eat more than if you ate on one plate containing these different types of food.

The central concept behind using smaller plates is that it fools your subconscious mind into thinking that you are not preventing yourself from eating.

When you prevent yourself from doing something, it's been found that it will become more desirable; the same applies when you start a diet because of the restrictions you impose on yourself.

Small plates will have your mind think that you have not set any restrictions on your eating habits because of the full plate served.

False ideas about food

A false idea is a belief that only exists in your mind and is not present in reality. For example, some people lack self-confidence because they have mistaken ideas about themselves; others fail to achieve their goals because they have false beliefs about success, while others have wrong ideas about food.

The following are examples of false ideas about food:

- I will forget my problems when I eat
- Food will make me feel happy even after I finish the meal
- Chocolate can fix me if I am down

The problem with these false ideas is that they keep you away from the real reasons that make you feel bad, making the problem worse.

If you have any of these beliefs or have similar thoughts, you should understand that food can never fix your mood forever. It can just do so for a few minutes or hours. Still, in the end, you will feel bad again, in addition to feeling guilty for overeating.

CHAPTER TWELVE
LOSING WEIGHT USING HYPNOSIS

Understanding the false beliefs that you might have about food is not enough on its own to make you lose weight or stop eating; you will still need a method to rid yourself of these false beliefs.

Sometimes people eat because they believe they cannot stop eating; at other times, people eat because they think that food can make them feel better. Every person have a unique set of beliefs about food consumption.

Still, in the end, they all share one specific thing, which is the inability to stop eating on account of these delusional beliefs!! Here, some people eat because they are trapped in thinking that they can't do anything about it.

It is one common theme with all bad habits, including emotional eating as people usually become haunted by a habit for years, just because of a false belief that prevents them from giving it up.

Hypnosis is a powerful therapy method mainly used to change a person's beliefs about a specific topic.

For example, suppose someone is firmly set that he could never give up chocolate. In that case, hypnosis can help him change that and eventually give it up.

On the other hand, suppose you are fully aware of yourself and your surroundings. In that case, your mind will always be filtering whatever you hear or see, aiming to prevent any unwanted ideas.

Those filters are called the conscious filters, and your conscious mind is that part of your brain responsible for them. Hypnosis mainly depends on silencing your conscious filters so that suggestions can pass directly to your subconscious.

For example, if you had a self-confidence problem and kept repeating phrases like "I am confident, I am confident" to yourself, you will end up feeling guilty because you will think that you are lying to yourself.

The same will happen if you kept telling yourself, "I don't like food" or "I won't eat chocolate again"; your conscious filters will discard these phrases because they are considered lies.

All hypnosis does is turn off those conscious filters so that suggestions can pass unfiltered to your subconscious mind.

Suppose a particular suggestion is kept bypassing your conscious filters.

In that case, it will end up being a solid belief stored in your subconscious mind. Now that you have understood the concept, the next part will be dealing with how you can hypnotize yourself to change the false beliefs you may have about food.

Hypnotizing yourself

Have you gone to sleep feeling very good about life but woke up in a terrible mood? While you are asleep, your conscious filters become turned off, which leaves your mood vulnerable to changes caused by any new ideas or beliefs entering your mind.

Suppose you go to sleep with the television left on; in that case, all that's being played will bypass your conscious filters and move directly to your subconscious mind as you sleep.

That's why you wake up in such a mood when you went to sleep feeling good; that could be on account of the horror movie that was playing when you drifted off to sleep.

Right before you go to sleep and right after you wake up, your conscious filters become unavailable; that's a natural state of hypnosis that can be used to suggesting new beliefs to yourself.

It also explains why you might wake up with some song at the back of your mind, and you'd keep singing it all day long without the slightest idea why or where you heard it; all that happened is that the song bypassed your conscious mind directly to your subconscious mind when your filters were not available.

Now here are the steps you need to put the new beliefs into your subconscious mind:

1) Keep repeating that belief over and over, all the while recording whatever it is you're saying. (For example, I hate chocolate)

2) While in bed, right before you sleep, start listening to the tape and allow yourself to fall asleep listening to it.

3) Do the same as soon as you wake up before you do anything else?

4) Within few weeks, if not days, the suggestions will turn into a belief

NOTE: Never uses a negative statement. You repeat this new belief to yourself as the subconscious mind doesn't consider negative words.

For example, something like "I won't eat chocolate again" is like telling your subconscious mind, "I will eat chocolate again." if this sounds weird, try now not imagining a green dog with six legs.

You see that the negatives are omitted, and you did imagine a green dog with six legs.

Below are some examples of beliefs you may use in your tape:

I like vegetables

I always like to eat healthy food

Chocolate is bad

The more I eat, the worse I'll feel.

Note that you are free to choose the new belief you want to implement as long as this belief deals with your existing false belief.

If you think that chocolates can solve your problems, then your thought could be, "the only way I can solve my problems is to take serious actions." as you can see, 'chocolates' were no mentioned.

Still, the belief itself convinced your subconscious mind that eating chocolate will not solve your existing problem.

Increasing your metabolic rate using hypnosis. If you were to find a way to increase your metabolic rate, you would lose weight without any significant effort. Fortunately, hypnosis allows you to do so.

For example, suppose you manage to convince your subconscious mind to think that you need to burn more calories. In that case, your metabolic rate will function faster.

The phrases used in such a case will focus on how your body burns calories and its rate.

Check the following examples:

"With every day that passes, my metabolic rate becomes faster; more and more calories are being burnt, and my weight is approaching the ideal weight."

As you receive such suggestions, you may start to notice that your breathing is becoming faster or that your heartbeat is going quicker.

It means that your subconscious mind accepted the suggestion and is working on it.

CHAPTER THIRTEEN

WEIGHT LOSS AND ANCHORS

Have you ever listened to a song that reminded you of a situation that happened long ago?

Have you ever smelled a perfume that reminded you of someone you know?

An anchor is when two events become linked with one another that one reminds you of the other.

Anchors usually take place when the two events start occurring together continuously over a particular time.

For example, if you keep listening to the same song when feeling happy, you will anchor a feeling of happiness to this song.

The real problem happens when you develop anchors of positive emotions and food; actually, most of those who overeat do so as food is anchored with happiness or satisfaction.

If you tend to eat a lot on birthdays, parties, and social gatherings, you may end up developing an anchor for the positive emotions you felt there with the food; the result will be recalling those positive emotions as soon as you eat.

In such a stressful world we live in, the presence of such anchors can drive people to try and recall their anchors as many times as they can, which in turn is translated to repetitive eating.

So one of the reasons you may be dissatisfied with your weight is anchors' presence for positive emotions associated with eating. So now we need to find a way to remove those anchors to eliminate our unwanted eating habits.

Back to the example of the song that reminds you of specific good memories; if you keep listening to the same music repeatedly without recalling that good memory, the music will lose its effect.

You won't feel happy again while listening to it. So if one of the two events kept occurring without the other's occurrence, then it will remove the anchor.

Now, how is it can we use this when it comes to food anchors? All you have to do is:

Not eat while feeling happy except if you're starving (people usually overeat at parties and birthdays when happy emotions are strong enough, thus creating a new anchor that is associated with eating)

When you are down, find other ways to comfort yourself other than eating. For example, instead of eating chocolate because you are depressed, try to run; you may end up anchoring running with happiness and so develop a new habit of running regularly.

Again, if you're starving, eat freely, but I am talking about the times when you eat because you are down and not when you are starving.

Where do you eat?
As you saw, anchors are formed when two events repeatedly occur at the same time. So now the question to be asked is this:

Where do I usually eat?

If you happen to be one of those people who eat all over the house, not in one specific place, and then you've just created an anchor of hunger that is associated with every single place in your house.

Think about it. Suppose you always take your meals in front of the television a few weeks later.

In that case, you will have formed an anchor that will get you hungry whenever you start watching the TV.

So you're not feeling hungry on account of that anchor and not because you're starving.

The same thing happens if you're used to drinking soda while sitting on your computer; even if you're not thirsty, you'll feel like something's missing till you get yourself your favorite drink.

Now the question is, how can I get rid of these anchors? You might have already guessed the answer.

Never eat except in the kitchen or a specific fixed place.

Never eat in front of the television.

Never eat while sitting in front of your computer.

Never eat while walking.

Now you might be wondering, what if I got hungry while watching my favorite show?

In this case, you have two options; the first is to go to your eating place and eat then get back to the show, part of which you'll have missed, while the second is to forget about eating, finish the show, then eat.

If you managed to keep that technique up for a few days, all those eating anchors would be uninstalled. Your hunger won't be spontaneously triggered as soon you did something you used to eat while doing it.

When a part of you resists the change

How many times have you overslept despite having had the alarm clock adjusted to waking you up earlier?

How many times have you kept on eating despite knowing that it was against your long-term weight loss goals?

How many times have you kept doing stuff without wanting to do it and ended up feeling very guilty about it?

It may seem odd that someone would keep at doing things that are against his best interest and then feel guilty about it; unfortunately, this is very common amongst people with inner conflicts.

When someone aims for a change, a part of him wants that, but another part of them resist that choice. If that change is, for example, a weight loss resolution, part of that person will be welcoming the change because it will make him more satisfied with his looks, while another faculty will be resisting the change as it prefers the status quo.

Just as conflicts can occur between people, they can occur within the same person when their conscious desires conflict with their unconscious ones.

Your conscious mind will be telling you, "we must lose weight, we must change our looks, and we must burn our fats," while your subconscious mind would be saying something like: "I hate exercising, I don't want to stop eating chocolate or drinking soda."

Such conflicts are prevalent, and the reasons behind them are very evident; part of you is attached to some beliefs that prevent it from accepting that change. In this case, you should first determine those limiting beliefs before initiating the change; else, this part will keep resisting.

Grab a comfortable seat, relax your muscles, and then ask yourself these questions: why am I refusing to give up food?

Why do I eat even when I don't want to?

What is the reason that is preventing me from being disciplined when it comes to food?

The more you ask yourself questions like these, the closer you will get to the limiting beliefs causing this inner conflict. Once you identify these limiting beliefs, one of the following two scenarios are bound to take place:

The first scenario: when the beliefs rise to the surface, you may discover that they were irrational and shouldn't have been there from the beginning.

For example, "I won't stop eating because food is the solution to my problems." suppose you're lucky to find such beliefs. In that case, your conscious mind will recognize that they should have been filtered earlier and will thus be discarded.

The second scenario: if you found a belief that can hardly be discarded, like "I adore chocolate," you can use the hypnosis technique mentioned above to change that belief.

Note that change can only be successful if both the conscious and the subconscious mind accept it; if only the conscious mind accepts it (like what happens in most situations), then a few days later, you will find that you have lost your motive and will thus head back to your starting point.

Weight loss and your body type

We don't have similar bodies, and each one of us has got a particular body type that requires a different way of dealing with when it comes to weight loss. The three major body types are the ectomorph, mesomorph, and endomorph.

The metabolic rate of an ectomorph is superfast, and that's why they are always slim. Even if an ectomorph gained some weight because of any other reason, losing this weight can take a few weeks without extra effort.

Mesomorphs have a naturally fit body even if they don't exercise. Mesomorphs are less vulnerable to weight gain than endomorphs because of the high energy level they possess.

Their lifestyle is usually full of action and vigorous exercises, which helps them stay in form even if they eat much.

You might have already guessed that endomorphs are the most vulnerable people to gain weight, their bodies are usually soft and round, and the rate at which they can lose weight is much slower than that of other body types.

If you are an endomorph, then the most important advice I have for you is not to compare yourself to others. For example, going to the gym with a mesomorph friend may cause you disappointment when he starts developing muscles much faster than you.

On the other hand, comparing yourself to an ectomorph will surely disappoint you because of their fast response to weight loss.

As an endomorph, you can develop muscles easier than the ectomorph; you should adjust your diet by focusing on proteins rather than carbohydrates and exercising regularly.

Being an endomorph means that your metabolic rate is a bit slow, which means that diet alone would never result in weight loss.

Therefore, in addition to changing your eating habits, you should follow the other instructions to increase the metabolic rate mentioned in this book.

The vital thing you must note is that people can fit somewhere between two body types; for example, if you are in between the endomorph and the mesomorph, then developing muscles and weight loss can give you a perfect body.

CHAPTER FOURTEEN

WEIGHT LOSS AND SELF DISCIPLINE

How many times have you started a diet then quit a few days later?

How many times have you failed to resist the urge to take a bite of a cake? How many times did you quit exercising a few weeks after you started?

Whenever you fail to sacrifice your short-term happiness for the sake of your long-term goals, then you should realize that you are dealing with a self-discipline problem.

Breaking any unwanted habit or sustaining any healthy habit can never happen unless you have a certain degree of self-discipline.

Since we are talking about lifestyle changes involving commitment for prolonged periods, you need to know how to develop discipline.

Unfortunately, people usually think that developing self-discipline means they will have to live their lives doing things they hate or avoiding stuff they like.

Still, the truth is that as soon as you commit to making a specific habit for three weeks, it will become a part of your lifestyle, and you won't need any extra effort to sustain it.

All the effort is needed when you first resist doing the things you were used to doing. Still, after that, your behavior will flow naturally. Of course, I am not saying that you will never return to your old habits after the three weeks, but your chance of returning will be a lot less.

You can develop self-discipline through only one thing, training. The more you resist the urge to do something, the more potent your self-discipline, and the more you fail to control your emotions and desires, the weaker your self-discipline becomes.

Usually, people make a big mistake when they try to develop self-discipline. They think that they should only be disciplined as long as circumstances are on their side.

For example, suppose someone started to develop the habit of running every day for 15 minutes, then on the fifth day. In that case, the weather conditions become bad.

Delaying his exercise to the next day would severely damage his self-discipline.

People usually think that they can forget about their self-discipline once or twice a week without affecting it. Still, the truth is that the more you let go of your discipline, the more you are weakening it.

The following are some popular ways of how people give themselves excuses to return to their old habits:

I am too tired today, so delaying exercising for tomorrow won't be a big problem

I had a stressful day today, and a piece of chocolate is what I deserve

The weather is cold today, and I should probably run tomorrow.

One more bite won't make a big difference; I'll be more careful tomorrow.

The summer is almost over, and nobody will see my belly until next year, so I will eat whatever I want.

Although the previous examples appear different, they are all rooted in the same false idea about developing self-discipline. If you want to have solid discipline, you need to know that the key to reaching it is a commitment, even if conditions were unfavourable.

It's even advised that you start to follow your new lifestyle or your new eating habit on a bad day.

If you managed to control yourself while feeling bad, maintaining yourself while feeling better would be cake.

Will power is not constant, but it changes with life events. Your willpower may be healthy on a good day.

Still, as soon as something terrible happens, your willpower can become weaker. Suppose you managed to resist food on a day where your willpower is feeble. In that case, you will be able to resist it in other situations.

Food addiction

Just as there is nicotine addiction and drug addiction, there is food addiction. I want you to try to eat a particular type of chocolate as soon as you wake every day for two weeks.

On the first day of the third week, I want you to wake up without eating the chocolate. You will probably find yourself craving for anything with the same ingredients as your chocolate, and nothing will satisfy you like eating a part of your usual daily chocolate. It can happen with any food or drink that you get used to and not just chocolate.

Your body, in this case, got used to certain nutrients with specific amounts. When you cut their supply, your body responded with this feeling of craving.

The good news is that if you resisted this craving feeling a few days later, you would wake up without finding yourself wanting to eat the same piece of chocolate.

So the question you should ask yourself now, are you eating because you are hungry, or is it just food addiction? If the answer is food addiction, you should gradually reduce such food intake until you get used to living without them.

Suppose you were addicted to peanut butter, you don't have to stop eating it all of a sudden, but you should reduce the amount you eat until you reach a certain amount that can fit into your healthy lifestyle.

After that, you can eat whatever food you like as long as the amount is acceptable.

Food addiction is one of the leading causes of prolonged obesity.

It's like the root of the tree mentioned before; if the basis of your eating habits is food addiction, then dieting will never help, nor will any other weight loss tips.

Food addiction could be the root cause of your eating habits, and to get rid of it, you need to know to get to the root cause.

People usually grow addicted to certain things when they feel bad for prolonged periods or prefer to escape their solved problems instead of dealing directly with them.

All of this happens on the unconscious level when the person is not aware that he is trying to escape; all he's aware of is that he is addicted to something.

People usually start to associate this addiction with other facts that are more acceptable to their subconscious minds, like:

- I love eating
- I am addicted to chocolate
- I can't resist peanut butter.

If you want to lose weight, then you should be brave enough to tear these masks apart so that you can see your real desires and the hidden agenda of your subconscious mind. Don't blame your subconscious mind for it; if you had been strong enough to face it initially, it wouldn't have been buried that deep.

Instead, your subconscious mind buried the real intentions deep because it knew that you wouldn't tolerate facing them directly.

To summarize food addiction in one word, it's "escape."

Getting addicted

Food addiction starts slowly and gradually so that the person never realizes that he is becoming addicted.

At first, the person feels terrible with hardly any kind of relief; he/she doesn't know what to do to get rid of those low feelings; he/she thus desperately start trying new things until he finds something that makes him feel better.

If eating is a relief, the person's mind forms an anchor, so food becomes anchored with happiness. Whenever the person feels down or wrong, he automatically starts eating to recall the anchor. A few months later, that person is landed with an obesity problem.

Suppose you want to prevent yourself from getting addicted to food. In that case, you should be aware of your emotions and problems to realize when you're eating to escape and when you're eating because you want to eat.

Mental effort & weight loss

Your brain cells consume double the energy required by any other cells in your body. That's why you may feel hungry after studying for a few hours or after a mentally demanding task. Boredom, sitting down without thinking of anything, and mental relaxation can be healthy, but too much of them can prevent your body from getting rid of extra energy, and the result may be weight gain.

If your current lifestyle doesn't involve any mentally demanding activities, you should implement a few changes. Learn something new, plan for your life or think of new ways to lose weight but don't just keep your mind empty most of the time.

Here, someone that lost weight on account of the mental effort said upon being asked for the reason:

"I was never on a diet; I neither stopped eating nor did I stop myself from eating anything. As soon as I started putting in 12 hours of work a day, I slowly started losing weight.

Over the months, the weight change was so significant that people kept asking me what I had done.

Everyone works, but I believe that the nature of my work which keeps my mind working for 12 straight hours, is the main reason."

Momentum eating

Try doing ten push-ups every morning for five days and watch what happens; by the third or fourth day, you'll most probably be able to finish something like over ten repetitions.

Whenever someone starts doing something, he/she gains a certain momentum that keeps him/her going at it till interrupted.

People who achieve hardly ever stop; they keep going for new goals and thus achieve more. Those who've managed to reach specific academic degrees don't stop there; they keep learning forever.

Those who start a typical habit keep at it till a significant change prevents them from continuing it.

Momentum is always perceived as a good thing, especially when looking at it through the previous examples. The real problem is when this momentum develops into a bad habit like overeating.

Suppose you were full when you decided to take a small bite off that delicious cake in front of you; the momentum that will arise out of this action will force you to keep eating more and more until you feel guilty.

You will only stop when the feelings of guilt are strong enough to counterbalance the momentum's strength.

Some people keep eating and feeling guilty until they end up broken over what they've done; that's one of the fundamental reasons behind binge eating, the momentum.

To prevent such momentum from forming, you have to do the following:

Understand that the next bite of the cake is not dangerous because of its calories but because of the momentum produced upon eating it

Know that there is nothing called "the last bite"; there are always more

Prevent yourself from taking the first bite if you're already full

Momentum is one of the most dangerous factors that could contribute to your weight; once it starts, a vicious endless cycle of eating is formed. When you start suffering from accumulated guilt, by then, it's already too late.

Interviews with formerly obese people

I have held interviews with some people who have lost significant weight and kept it off for at least one year. I have selected the most important phrases used in the interview so you can know about the issues that dramatically affected their weight.

Below are their comments:

'Diet fails because people start dieting just before the summer, so they'd fit into summer clothes and then forget about it when the winter comes.

Weight loss is effortless; all you need is a permanent lifestyle change, not just a course before the summer comes.

"Y.K _ from being overweight to being slim."

I never used to exercise, but then one day I started exercising daily and still do. I never stopped eating anything; I just ate healthier food and reduced the quantities I ate. Diets fail when people feel that they are dieting. The correct thing to do is eat whatever you want while keeping up the exercise. Having a long-term perspective is the key; your goal should not be losing weight this month but maintaining a healthy lifestyle.

"Anonymous- from being extremely overweight to being super fit."

What I did was start exercising; I then committed myself to do so every day until it became a part of my lifestyle. I didn't stop eating what I liked but just started adding healthy food to my diet; that left less space for junk food in my life.

"H.A- from being obese to having an athletic body."

As you can see, all of them are almost saying the same thing despite not knowing anything of the book's content or hearing from one another talk. Reaching an ideal weight is not a challenging task at all; you need to do the following practical steps:

1) On a piece of paper, write down five lifestyle changes you are ready to commit to forever.

2) Commit to these lifestyle changes till they become a part of your life

3) Know that you aren't going to have an ideal weight in a week or two but that you are following a long term approach that is much more effective than such a short term approach

4) If you got used to these lifestyle changes, add another five lifestyle changes and start committing to them.

5) Be patient until you notice the effect

Setting clear goals

You should set clear goals for losing weight. People who undergo a diet usually feel guilty or even depressed because they didn't manage to reach the impossible target they had set for themselves.

When setting a goal, make sure that it can be measured to monitor your progress. Avoid setting goals like these:

- I will be in shape by the end of the summer
- I will look like a model
- I will have a perfect body

Such goals can only lead you to depression because they are unclear and undefined. The correct thing would be specifying the exact amount of weight you want to lose during the summer or the next few months.

Make sure also that your goal is realistic. You can't just set a goal of losing 100 pounds in 2 months; again, you will become depressed.

As you have already learned, your mood is one of the most substantial factors that can affect your weight, and you don't want another mood swing or another depression that results from unmet goals because it can ruin your weight loss plans.

Are you obese?

Many girls follow specific diets, even slim ones!! I know several girls who are super skinny yet think that they are obese.

For some reason, those people have built an incorrect self-image that makes them believe they are overweight.

What makes it even worse is that your mind start looking for incorrect evidence to support your false self-image.

For example, one of these girls may go shopping and buy the smallest shirt in the shop; then, she thinks that she is overweight after trying it. Her subconscious mind made her choose the small shirt to prove to her that she is fat.

Your subconscious mind doesn't care about the validity of the beliefs you carry; it just tries to prove them by letting you only notice things that support them.

You must ask yourself a crucial question before thinking about weight loss, "Am I really in need of a diet, or do I just need to change my mental self-image?"

Why are you stalling?

While surveying some of the people who want to lose weight, I found that lots of them are well educated about some of the facts that may help in weight loss, like the importance of exercising, the importance of vegetables, and other relevant factors.

I was amazed at that realization, and I feel bad for them because the body doesn't care about what we know; it only cares and is affected by what we apply.

How can you be familiar with that kind of information and choose not to put it to use? What's keeping you from starting right now?

Weight loss is a straightforward process that can apply with hardly any difficulties, given that you follow all the pieces of advice given in this book, in addition to anything else you may already know.

If you are serious about weight loss, then don't turn this into another book you have read without any effort to apply the information given through it.

Some of the techniques provided are very powerful, but people have never tried using them!! You have now reached the end of the book.

Have you prepared the picture that you are going to hang everywhere in your house? If not, what are you stalling?

All the advice provided in the book is practical and can be applied without any difficulties; don't keep on blaming the reasons behind your weight when you're the one to be blamed for not doing anything about it.

You will never lose weight by reading e-books and online articles; you need to apply what you're reading.

Start now, or else nothing will change.

Summary

As you can see, your current weight reflects your lifestyle, resulting from your eating habits, exercising habits, and other habits.

Permanent changes to your lifestyle are the key to a permanent change in your weight.

All you have to do is change the factors listed above, then commit to these new behaviors, and sooner or later, it will be reflected on your weight.

That's why lots of diet programs fail because they only focus on nutrients and food intake without paying attention to the full picture.

About the author

Kristine Knutson is a family therapist that lives in the United States, she is passionate in helping people enjoy healthy and meaningful lives. She is excited to contribute her knowledge and expertise so people can live the best life possible.

Her books present evidence based principles in a ready-to-apply format, so people can lose weight, give up addictions, fight off and prevent disease among others.

This book is the course material for my highly successful 'bad habit breakup accountability program' where I help people dissolve all the obstacles they encounter in breaking a bad habit. I also help them create a habit replacement alternative for their bad habits.

You can send her a mail drkristineknutson@gmail.com

Other titles by the author include:

Lose weight This Way Not That Way: Lose weight without dieting, even while you sleep and keep it off forever

Break Any Bad Habit This Way Not That Way: Quit any addiction, break bad habits without will power